PELVIC INFLAMMATORY DISEASE (PID) RECIPES FOR NEWLY DIAGNOSED

Wholesome Meal Ideas Tailored To Target Inflammation, Combat Symptoms, Boost Immunity, And Restore Balance In The Body

DR. ERIC TRISTAN

CONTENTS

DISCLAIMER

The information provided in this book, is intended for informational purposes only. The content is not intended to be a substitute for professional medical advice, diagnosis, or treatment. Always seek the advice of your physician or other qualified health provider with any questions you may have regarding a medical condition. Never disregard professional medical advice or delay in seeking it because of something you have read in this book.

The author of this book has made reasonable efforts to ensure that the information provided is accurate and up-to-date at the time of publication. However, the author makes no representations or warranties of any kind, express or implied, about the completeness, accuracy, reliability, suitability, or availability of the information contained within these pages.

Any reliance you place on the information provided in this book is strictly at your own risk. The author shall not be liable for any loss, injury, or damage arising from the use of this book or the information contained herein.

The mention or reference to any individuals, products, websites, organizations, or other names within this book does not imply endorsement by the author. The inclusion of such references is solely for informational purposes and does not constitute an endorsement or recommendation.

Furthermore, the author disclaims any association or affiliation with any individuals, products, websites, organizations, or other names mentioned in this book.

It is important to consult with a qualified healthcare professional before making any dietary or lifestyle changes, especially if you have a medical condition. Each individual's health situation is unique, and what works for one person may not work for another.

Again, the information provided in this book is not intended to diagnose, treat, cure, or prevent any disease or health condition. Always seek the advice of a physician or other qualified health provider regarding any medical questions or concerns you may have.

Thank you for your understanding and for taking the necessary precautions when considering the information presented in this book.

ABOUT THIS BOOK

"Pelvic Inflammatory Disease (PID) Recipes" is an essential resource for those who are navigating the intricacies of PID. It provides a thorough guide to nutritional management that is specifically designed to address the needs of this particular health condition. This book begins with a perceptive "Introduction to Pelvic Inflammatory Disease (PID)," which offers a fundamental comprehension of the condition. It examines the complexities of PID, investigates its etiology, and illuminates the significance of nutrition in the management of the condition. This paper elaborates on the critical significance of a PID-friendly diet and provides clear and practical guidelines to assist individuals in developing a nutritionally sound approach to their health.

This book makes a systematic progression, offering a diverse selection of informative material that encompasses breakfast, lunch, and dinner recipes specifically designed to aid in the management of

PID as well as nutrient-dense foods that are appropriate for this condition. This comprehensive approach of the dietary recommendations is emphasized by the provision of refreshment options and beverages that are made specifically for individuals with PID. Furthermore, this book discusses foods that individuals with PID should avoid, offering crucial advice on how to circumvent potential triggers.

The integration of sample meal plans for PID promotes practicality by facilitating the smooth transition of the recommended dietary modifications into daily life. Anti-inflammatory substances, culinary herbs, and seasonings are incorporated to augment the nutritional strategies that have been delineated. Furthermore, this book expands its reach beyond merely listing recipes by providing insightful advice on meal planning and preparation utilizing PID. The statement recognizes the significance of incorporating lifestyle changes into one's routine to enhance pelvic health, as well as the correlation between dietary choices and general welfare.

Moreover, this publication titled "Pelvic Inflammatory Disease (PID) Recipes" acknowledges the importance of seeking expert advice and promotes the idea of working in tandem with nutritionists and dietitians. By incorporating a dedicated section addressing frequently asked questions (FAQs) about PID and nutrition, the information presented is more easily comprehensible and applicable.

Fundamentally, this book serves as an indispensable resource, facilitating the transition from theoretical medical comprehension to tangible dietary application by providing a comprehensive strategy for managing PID via well-informed dietary decisions.

CHAPTER ONE

An Overview Of Pelvic Inflammatory Disease

Pelvic Inflammatory Disease (PID) is a critical medical condition that impacts the reproductive system of women. It manifests when the infection progresses to the ovaries, fallopian tubes, and uterus, which are all components of the upper genital tract.

PID, which is commonly induced by sexually transmitted infections (STIs) such as chlamydia and gonorrhea, can result in significant repercussions if untreated. These may comprise chronic pelvic discomfort, infertility, and an elevated likelihood of ectopic pregnancy.

PID results from the upward migration of microbes from the cervix or vagina to the upper reproductive organs. Symptoms frequently observed include pelvic pain, irregular vaginal discharge, fever, and discomfort during sexual activity. Prompt treatment and early diagnosis are essential for preventing long-term complications.

Comprehending PID And Its Origins

PID is predominantly caused by microorganisms ascending from the lower reproductive tract to the upper organs. Although Chlamydia trachomatis and Neisseria gonorrhoeae are frequently implicated pathogens, additional bacteria, including those present in the typical vaginal flora, may also play a role. A history of sexually transmitted infections, multiple sexual partners, youth, and intrauterine device use are all risk factors for PID.

Upon infiltration of the upper reproductive organs, the bacteria induce inflammation and inflict harm upon the vulnerable tissues. Such complications may include adhesions, abscesses, scar tissue formation, and compromised reproductive function. PID can have ramifications that transcend the immediate infection, potentially exerting an influence on fertility and reproductive health in its entirety.

PID prevention requires the use of condoms, routine STI screenings, and prompt treatment of any infections that are detected, among other safe sexual practices. Individuals must be informed of the dangers and repercussions of STIs to reduce the incidence and severity of PID.

Nutritional Importance In The Management Of PID

The function of nutrition in the management of PID, support of the immune system, and promotion of overall health is crucial. Healing and recovery are dependent upon proper nutrition, particularly in the case of infections and inflammation. Adhering to a healthy diet can aid in the alleviation of symptoms, the reduction of inflammation, and the enhancement of the body's immune system.

In response to the energy demands of the immune system and the healing process, the body's nutritional needs may increase during an episode of PID. Important nutrients for immune function and tissue repair, including vitamins, minerals, antioxidants, and protein, are found in a well-balanced diet.

PID-Friendly Dietary Recommendations

Embracing a PID-friendly diet necessitates the selection of foods that promote cellular recovery and diminish inflammation. Consider the following general guidelines:

1. Incorporate anti-inflammatory food sources, such as fruits and vegetables, fatty fish (e.g., mackerel and salmon), almonds, and seeds, into one's diet. These nutrients may aid in the reduction of reproductive organ inflammation.

2. Select whole cereals such as quinoa, brown rice, and whole wheat, as they are rich in essential nutrients, fiber, and complex carbohydrates.

3. Lean Proteins: Opt for lean protein sources, including tofu, poultry, fish, and legumes. Protein is essential for immune function and tissue repair.

4. To promote digestive health, include probiotic-rich foods in your diet, such as fermented vegetables, yogurt, and kefir. A correlation exists between a healthy intestinal microbiome and immune function as a whole.

5. Maintain proper hydration by ingesting a sufficient quantity of water. Supporting hydration is essential for optimal body functioning and contaminant elimination.

6. Reduce Consumption of Processed Foods: Adhere to a restricted diet of refined carbohydrates, sweetened munchies, and processed foods. These have the potential to exacerbate inflammation and have adverse effects on overall health.

7. It is advisable to restrict the consumption of alcohol and caffeine to a moderate level, as excessive ingestion has the potential to impair immune function and worsen inflammation.

Foods Rich In Nutrients For PID

Specific nutrients are critical for the management of PID and the promotion of recovery. Complement your diet with the following nutrient-dense foods:

1. Vitamin C, which is present in broccoli, citrus fruits, strawberries, and bell peppers, aids in tissue repair and immune system support.

2. Zinc: Foods abundant in zinc, including lean meats, nuts, seeds, and legumes, possess anti-inflammatory and wound-healing properties.

3. Omega-3 oily Acids: Walnuts, flaxseeds, and oily fish (such as salmon and sardines) are rich in omega-3 fatty acids, which possess anti-inflammatory properties.

4. Vitamin E: Avocados, nuts, seeds, and spinach are all excellent sources of vitamin E, an antioxidant that strengthens the immune system.

5. Incorporate lean protein sources such as chicken, fish, tofu, and legumes into your diet to aid in immune function and tissue repair.

6. Fiber is present in fruits, vegetables, whole cereals, and legumes; it aids in the elimination of impurities from the body and promotes digestive health.

7. Probiotic foods comprise kefir, kimchi, yogurt, and sauerkraut, all of which contain beneficial microorganisms that promote digestive health and immunity as a whole.

Managing PID, in summary, necessitates a comprehensive strategy encompassing medical intervention, modifications to one's lifestyle, and appropriate nutrition.

Incorporating a PID-friendly diet, which is abundant in anti-inflammatory and vital nutrients, can significantly contribute to facilitating the body's recovery and mitigating the likelihood of complications linked to PID.

CHAPTER TWO

An Examination Of Pelvic Inflammatory Disease (PID): A Nutritional Approach To Management

Pelvic Inflammatory Disease (PID) is a pathological state characterized by inflammation and possible chronic impairment of the female reproductive organs.

It is commonly caused by the transmission of bacterial infections, which frequently originate from sexually transmitted diseases (STIs) such as chlamydia or gonorrhea. A multifaceted approach, including medical intervention, is required to manage PID; however, nutrition is of critical importance in promoting the body's restoration.

This book examines particular recipes and dietary considerations associated with each meal to assist those with PID.

Breakfast that is rich in nutrients is a critical dietary component for individuals diagnosed with PID. By consuming foods abundant in antioxidants, vitamins, and minerals, one can reduce inflammation and strengthen the immune system. Consider making a smoothie concoction for brunch. Blend frozen berries, spinach, Greek yogurt, and a dash of almond milk. Nuts, seeds, and sliced fruits are used to add texture and nutritional value. Toast made with whole grains, avocado, and poached eggs is an additional option. Eggs contain protein and avocado contains healthful lipids, both of which are essential for maintaining overall health. Moreover, the fiber content of whole grains promotes digestive health and contributes to a well-balanced diet.

Lunch Suggestions For People With PID: Saturating And Inspiring

Consider consuming dishes that are nourishing and fulfilling for lunch. A vegetable and quinoa salad accompanied by seared chicken is an outstanding option. In addition to being a complete protein, quinoa is an excellent source of numerous vitamins and minerals. Lean protein, which is added to grilled chicken, promotes muscle health. Consider substituting lentils into a serving of vegetable broth. Lentils provide the body with protein and iron, both of which aid in the healing process. The hydrating properties of the bouillon in the soup are crucial for individuals diagnosed with PID. Complement the meal with whole grain crackers or bread on the side for a gratifying and energizing lunch.

Dinner Recipes To Assist In PID Management: Vegetables And Proteins In Balance

Dinner provides the chance to achieve a protein-vegetable balance, which aids in the management of PID. Salmon grilled alongside roasted sweet potatoes and steamed broccoli constitutes a palatable and healthful alternative. Salmon is rich in anti-inflammatory omega-3 fatty acids, whereas sweet potatoes are a source of micronutrients and complex carbohydrates.

Consider brown rice stir-fried with chickpeas and vegetables as a vegetarian alternative. The high protein and fiber content of chickpeas aids in digestion and satiety. An assortment of nutrients is provided by the stir-fry's assortment of vegetables, which contributes to overall health.

Snack Alternatives For Individuals Managing PID: Optimal And Inspiring Selections

It is essential to select nutritious refreshments to sustain energy levels and aid in the body's recuperation throughout the day. Berry-topped Greek yogurt with a drizzle of honey constitutes a scrumptious and nutritionally rich refreshment. Berry concentrates microorganisms, which are known to support digestive health, while Greek yogurt is an excellent source of antioxidants.

Additionally, a fistful of assorted nuts and seeds can be a snack. Nuts and seeds comprise vital nutrients, such as vitamin E and omega-3 fatty acids, which are responsible for their anti-inflammatory properties.

Nevertheless, moderation is crucial in light of their caloric content.

Included Beverages In A PID-Focused Diet: Healing And Hydration

Constant hydration is of the utmost importance for those with PID, as it facilitates the elimination of impurities and promotes general well-being. Chamomile and ginger tea are examples of herbal beverages that possess soothing and anti-inflammatory properties. Furthermore, maintaining proper hydration with water infused with cucumber, lemon, or mint slices not only imparts a revitalizing element but also supplies vital fluids.

It is recommended to limit consumption of caffeine and alcohol, as these substances have the potential to worsen inflammation and disrupt the body's natural healing mechanisms. To satisfy one's hydration requirements, decaffeinated herbal beverages or plain flavored water should be chosen.

In summary, the management of PID necessitates a holistic strategy, with nutrition serving as an indispensable component in facilitating the recovery process. By integrating foods that are rich in nutrients into their daily diets, individuals have the potential to enhance their general health and potentially mitigate certain symptoms that are linked to PID. It is advisable to seek guidance from a registered dietitian or a healthcare professional to customize these dietary recommendations according to personal preferences and requirements.

The Significance Of Nutrition In The Management Of Pelvic Inflammatory Disease (PID)

A condition affecting the female reproductive organs, Pelvic Inflammatory Disease (PID) is frequently caused by the ascending spread of bacteria from the cervix and vagina to the uterus, fallopian tubes, and ovaries. Although medical intervention is of utmost importance in the treatment of PID, incorporating a supportive nutritional approach can be highly beneficial in symptom management and the promotion of general health. This book examines the correlation between nutrition and peptic ulcer inflammation (PID), with an emphasis on meal plans that incorporate anti-inflammatory ingredients, foods to exclude, and the application of culinary seasonings and condiments.

CHAPTER THREE

A Compensatory Dietary Approach To Pelvic Inflammatory Disease: A List Of Foods To Avoid

Instability in the body can be influenced by dietary decisions; therefore, individuals with PID must be particularly mindful of particular foods that may worsen symptoms or impede the healing process. Restrict the consumption of foods that are rich in sugar, refined carbohydrates, and saturated fats, as doing so may compromise the immune system and promote inflammation.

1. A diet high in refined carbohydrates and sugar may contribute to heightened inflammation. Minimal consumption of processed foods, sweetened munchies, and beverages is recommended to mitigate the risk of hyperglycemia. In the same way that refined carbohydrates, which are present in white bread and pasta, can contribute to inflammation, whole grains should be substituted for them.

2. Saturated lipids, including those found in high concentrations in red meat and full-fat dairy products, have the potential to promote inflammation and hinder the body's regenerative processes. As a potentially healthier alternative, lean protein sources such as poultry, fish, and plant-based proteins may be preferred.

3. Caffeine and alcohol have the potential to induce dehydration in the body, which may worsen pelvic pain and discomfort. It is recommended to restrict the consumption of caffeinated beverages and alcohol to promote proper hydration and overall health. PID patients can establish a groundwork for recovery and symptom control by refraining from these inflammatory triggers.

Sample PID Meal Plans: Nutritional Balance For Optimal Health

A well-rounded diet can reduce inflammation and support the immune system, making the development of balanced meal plans crucial for individuals managing PID. Let the subsequent illustrative meal plans serve as an initial reference:

Day 1:

• Greek yogurt topped with berries and a pinch of chia seeds for breakfast.

• A handful of hazelnuts as a snack.

• Grilled chicken salad accompanied by cherry tomatoes, mixed greens, and olive oil vinaigrette for lunch.

Snack: apple slices spread with almond butter.

Baked salmon served with quinoa and stewed broccoli for supper.

Day 2:

• Oatmeal garnished with banana slices and a drizzle of honey for breakfast.

• Hummus-topped carrot and cucumber spears as a snack.

• Lentil soup accompanied by whole-grain bread for lunch.

• Greek yogurt parfait with granola and fresh fruit serves as a snack.

Tofu stir-fried with brown rice and an assortment of vegetables for supper.

The meal plans emphasize the consumption of whole foods, lean proteins, and an assortment of vibrant fruits and vegetables, thereby supplying the body with vital nutrients that aid in its recovery.

Integrating Anti-Inflammatory Components:

The integration of anti-inflammatory components into one's dietary regimen may amplify the body's capacity to regulate symptoms associated with PID. Consider including the nutrient-dense dishes listed below:

1. Salmon, mackerel, and sardines are excellent sources of omega-3 fatty acids, which possess anti-

inflammatory characteristics. These may aid in inflammation reduction and general health promotion.

2. Brightly colored vegetables, such as kale, spinach, and bell peppers, are rich in vitamins and antioxidants that reduce inflammation and strengthen the immune system.

3. Antioxidants are abundant in raspberries, blueberries, and strawberries; they aid in the fight against inflammation and strengthen the body's natural defenses.

4. Curcumin, which is present in turmeric, is widely recognized for its potent anti-inflammatory attributes. The consumption of turmeric beverages or the addition of turmeric to food can be beneficial.

5. Antioxidants and polyphenols, which are found in green tea, may aid in inflammation reduction and promote overall health.

Proactive contributors to the well-being and symptom management of individuals with PID may benefit from the inclusion of these anti-inflammatory ingredients in their regimens.

Herbs And Spices Used In The Kitchen To Improve Flavor And Health Benefits For PID

Herbs and seasonings used in the kitchen not only impart flavor to food but also provide numerous health benefits. PID patients may find the following botanicals and ingredients to be especially beneficial:

1. Ginger, which is recognized for its anti-inflammatory attributes, may be incorporated into stir-fries, stews, or beverages to augment flavor and offer possible health advantages.

2. Garlic possesses anti-inflammatory and antimicrobial properties. Fresh garlic added to food may strengthen the body's natural defenses.

3. Cinnamon, which has been associated with potential anti-inflammatory properties, can be utilized as a garnish for a variety of dishes or blended into beverages to enhance their taste.

4. Basil: Anti-inflammatory compounds are present in basil, which can be utilized to impart flavor to pasta, salads, and sauces.

5. Antioxidant-rich cilantro imparts a zesty taste to food preparations. As a garnish or in salads and salsas, it is a versatile ingredient.

In summary, the integration of a deliberate nutritional strategy with medical interventions for Pelvic Inflammatory Disease can serve as a complementary approach. Through the implementation of a balanced meal plan, the exclusion of inflammatory foods, the integration of culinary herbs and seasonings, and the incorporation of anti-inflammatory ingredients, individuals with PID can gain the ability to advocate for their health and well-being. It is recommended that individuals consistently seek guidance from healthcare professionals or nutritionists to tailor dietary recommendations to their specific health requirements.

Palpitas Inflammatory Disease (PID): Exploring The Role Of Nutrition

Pelvic Inflammatory Disease (PID) is a pathological state that impacts the ovaries and uterus and is frequently attributed to bacterial infections that ascend from the cervix or vagina to the uterus. Although medical intervention is of utmost importance in the management of PID, incorporating a nutrition-focused approach can enhance overall health and facilitate the body's recovery.

CHAPTER FOUR

Recipes For Pelvic Inflammatory Disease (PID)

A healthy diet is an absolute necessity for those who are afflicted with PID. The immune system can be fortified and the body can obtain the essential resources for recuperation from nutrient-dense foods. The following recipes are PID-friendly and emphasize medicinal ingredients:

1. Blended Anti-Inflammatory Juice:

• Components:

• One cup of a variety of berries (strawberries, raspberries, and blueberries)

• One-half cup Greek yogurt

• One teaspoonful of chia seed meal

One-half teaspoon honey

• One-half cup almond milk

Compile these components in a blender to produce a scrumptious and nourishing smoothie that is laden with anti-inflammatory and antioxidant properties.

2. Quinoa and Salmon Bowl:

• Components:

• Salmon fillet grilled

One cup of quinoa, boiled

• Broccoli and spinach steamed

One tablespoon of olive oil is required.

• Lemon juice added for taste

By containing protein, fiber, and omega-3 fatty acids, this serving promotes a healthy, well-balanced diet.

3. Legume Soup Infused with Turmeric:

• Components:

(1) cup cooked legumes

2. Two diced vegetables

• One diced onion

• Two minced cloves of garlic

One-eighth teaspoon turmeric

Broth composed of vegetables

Due to the anti-inflammatory properties of turmeric, individuals with PID may find this soup to be a soothing and curative alternative.

Suggestions For Planning And Preparing Meals With PID

1. Place an Emphasis on Whole Foods: Choose unadulterated, whole foods that are abundant in antioxidants, vitamins, and minerals. Aside from aiding in recovery, fresh fruits, vegetables, lean proteins, and whole grains all contribute to overall health.

2. Maintaining proper hydration is vital for overall health and can aid in inflammation management. Incorporate into your daily regimen water, botanical

teas, and infused water made with cucumber or citrus fruit segments.

3. It is essential to maintain a well-balanced macronutrient intake, which includes proteins, carbohydrates, and healthful lipids. This contributes to energy maintenance and strengthens the body's restorative mechanisms.

4. Engage in mindful dining by cultivating the practice of savoring every mouthful and remaining attuned to the signals of hunger and fullness. This method has the potential to improve nutrient digestion and assimilation.

5. It is advisable to restrict the intake of processed and high-sugar foods, as they have the potential to exacerbate inflammation and impede the recovery process.

Alterations To One's Lifestyle To Promote Pelvic Health

In addition to dietary adjustments, specific adjustments to one's lifestyle may support the enhancement of pelvic health in individuals afflicted with PID. The following are some suggestions:

1. Consistent Physical Activity: Maintain a routine of moderate exercise to enhance circulation and mitigate inflammation. Seek guidance from a healthcare professional to ascertain appropriate exercise regimens.

2. The management of chronic stress has the potential to adversely affect pelvic health. Integrate into your daily regimen stress-relieving practices such as yoga, meditation, or deep breathing exercises.

3. It is essential to prioritize adequate sleep to facilitate the body's natural healing process. Adequate sleep is critical for immune function and general health.

4. Adopt safer sexual practices to mitigate the risk of bacterial infections that have the potential to result in PID reoccurring. Communicate candidly with your partner and consistently employ protective measures.

5. Consistent Check-ups: Establish a routine schedule for check-ups with your healthcare provider to oversee the condition of your pelvis and promptly attend to any concerns that may arise.

Consulting With Dietitians And Nutritionists For Professional Guidance

In the management of PID, it can be advantageous to consult with nutritionists and dietitians for professional guidance. Personalized nutrition plans that are customized to individual requirements and health conditions can be developed by these specialists. They can be of the following assistance:

1. Tailored Nutrition Plans: Dietitians and nutritionists possess the expertise to formulate individualized meal plans that precisely correspond

to the nutritional needs of those coping with PID. This approach promotes holistic and encouraging healing.

2. Education and Guidance: Experts in this domain possess the ability to impart knowledge regarding the correlation between nutrition and pelvic health, thereby enabling individuals to make knowledgeable dietary decisions that positively impact their overall health.

3. Monitoring and Modifications: Consistent consultations allow nutritionists to assess progress and implement required modifications to the nutrition regimen. This adaptive methodology guarantees continuous assistance throughout the person's health trajectory.

4. Nutritionists possess the ability to detect and rectify any nutrient deficiencies that could be impeding the process of recuperation. The need for supplementation may be advised in certain circumstances.

FAQs (Frequently Asked Questions) Regarding PID And Nutrition

Can specific foods exacerbate symptoms of PID?

A1: Although no universally applicable "PID diet" exists, specific food items might worsen inflammation. Caffeine, refined foods, and sugary treats should be restricted, as they may contribute to inflammation.

Q2: Do particular nutrients contribute to the maintenance of pelvic health?

A2: Indeed, antioxidants, vitamin C, omega-3 fatty acids, and zinc all contribute to the maintenance of pelvic health. These nutrients are present in an assortment of fruits, vegetables, and lean proteins.

Can weight management affect PID?

A3: Sustaining a healthy weight influences pelvic health positively, which is an aspect of overall health.

Being overweight can be a contributing factor to inflammation; therefore, maintaining a healthy weight and engaging in consistent physical activity can provide support.

Q4: What dietary modifications should I make during a flare-up of a PID?

A4: Concentrate on readily digestible foods during a flare-up. Smoothies, stews, and well-cooked vegetables should be considered. Avoid foods that could aggravate the digestive system and maintain adequate hydration.

Q5: Is supplementation acceptable to consume while on PID?

A5: It is advisable to seek guidance from a healthcare professional before incorporating any supplements into your regimen. If deficiencies are detected, they may recommend supplements after evaluating your particular requirements.

In summary, individuals afflicted with Pelvic Inflammatory Disease must embrace a comprehensive strategy encompassing nourishing meal plans, adjustments to one's lifestyle, and access to expert advice.

By incorporating these components into one's daily routine, one can enhance overall wellness and facilitate the body's recuperative mechanisms. It is advisable to consistently seek personalized advice from healthcare professionals regarding one's particular health condition.

Conclusion

As a result, the integration of a targeted dietary regimen may serve as a beneficial supplementary strategy in the management of pelvic inflammatory disease. Although recipes cannot serve as a substitute for medical intervention, they can be beneficial in facilitating recovery and promoting overall health.

Emphasizing consuming an anti-inflammatory diet, which includes fruits, vegetables, and omega-3 fatty acids, could potentially aid in the mitigation of inflammation that is linked to PID.

Prioritize nutrient-dense ingredients recognized for their anti-inflammatory properties when developing recipes for PID. Compounds found in garlic, turmeric, and ginger, for instance, may possess antimicrobial and anti-inflammatory properties.

The incorporation of these ingredients into recipes may improve the health of individuals with PID. Furthermore, it is critical to prioritize gastrointestinal health, as recent studies indicate a potential correlation between the microbiota in the intestine and the health of the pelvis.

It is of the utmost importance that individuals diagnosed with PID seek guidance from healthcare professionals to ensure that any dietary modifications are by their comprehensive treatment regimen.

Furthermore, individualized nutrition counseling can effectively target particular requirements and factors to be taken into account.

In essence, PID remedies ought to be perceived as an adjunctive component to traditional medical practices, to facilitate the body's recuperative mechanisms and augment general welfare.

THE END